Cambridge Elements

Elements in Emergency Neurosurgery
edited by
Nihal Gurusinghe
Lancashire Teaching Hospital NHS Trust
Peter Hutchinson
University of Cambridge, Society of British Neurological Surgeons and Royal College of Surgeons of England
Ioannis Fouyas
Royal College of Surgeons of Edinburgh
Naomi Slator
North Bristol NHS Trust
Ian Kamaly-Asl
Royal Manchester Children's Hospital
Peter Whitfield
University Hospitals Plymouth NHS Trust

INTRACRANIAL ABSCESS IN ADULTS

See Yung Phang
Institute of Neurological Sciences, Glasgow
William Taylor
Institute of Neurological Sciences, Glasgow

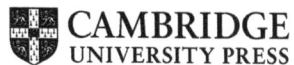

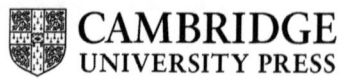

Shaftesbury Road, Cambridge CB2 8EA, United Kingdom

One Liberty Plaza, 20th Floor, New York, NY 10006, USA

477 Williamstown Road, Port Melbourne, VIC 3207, Australia

314–321, 3rd Floor, Plot 3, Splendor Forum, Jasola District Centre, New Delhi – 110025, India

103 Penang Road, #05–06/07, Visioncrest Commercial, Singapore 238467

Cambridge University Press is part of Cambridge University Press & Assessment, a department of the University of Cambridge.

We share the University's mission to contribute to society through the pursuit of education, learning and research at the highest international levels of excellence.

www.cambridge.org
Information on this title: www.cambridge.org/9781009487511
DOI: 10.1017/9781009487498

© See Yung Phang and William Taylor 2025

This publication is in copyright. Subject to statutory exception and to the provisions of relevant collective licensing agreements, no reproduction of any part may take place without the written permission of Cambridge University Press & Assessment.

When citing this work, please include a reference to the DOI 10.1017/9781009487498

First published 2025

A catalogue record for this publication is available from the British Library

ISBN 978-1-009-48751-1 Paperback
ISSN 2755-0656 (online)
ISSN 2755-0648 (print)

Cambridge University Press & Assessment has no responsibility for the persistence or accuracy of URLs for external or third-party internet websites referred to in this publication and does not guarantee that any content on such websites is, or will remain, accurate or appropriate.

For EU product safety concerns, contact us at Calle de José Abascal, 56, 1°, 28003 Madrid, Spain, or email eugpsr@cambridge.org

Every effort has been made in preparing this Element to provide accurate and up-to-date information which is in accord with accepted standards and practice at the time of publication. Although case histories are drawn from actual cases, every effort has been made to disguise the identities of the individuals involved. Nevertheless, the authors, editors and publishers can make no warranties that the information contained herein is totally free from error, not least because clinical standards are constantly changing through research and regulation. The authors, editors and publishers therefore disclaim all liability for direct or consequential damages resulting from the use of material contained in this Element. Readers are strongly advised to pay careful attention to information provided by the manufacturer of any drugs or equipment that they plan to use.

Intracranial Abscess in Adults

Elements in Emergency Neurosurgery

DOI: 10.1017/9781009487498
First published online: December 2025

See Yung Phang
Institute of Neurological Sciences, Glasgow

William Taylor
Institute of Neurological Sciences, Glasgow

Author for correspondence: See Yung Phang, Seeyung.phang2@nhs.scot

Abstract: Adult cerebral infections are a common neurosurgical emergency presentation in the UK. This Element provides a comprehensive guide for clinicians, detailing the epidemiology, aetiology, and risk factors associated with the various types of cerebral infections, including cerebral abscess, subdural empyema, epidural abscess, and cranial fungal and parasitic infections. The clinical presentation, diagnostic methods, and treatment options, including surgical and antibiotic management, are discussed. Emphasis is placed on the importance of early diagnosis and tailored treatment plans. Flow diagrams summarizing the management of cerebral infections are also provided in this Element.

Keywords: adult, cranial, infections, investigation, management

© See Yung Phang and William Taylor 2025

ISBNs: 9781009487511 (PB), 9781009487498 (OC)
ISSNs: 2755-0656 (online), 2755-0648 (print)

Contents

Adult Cerebral Abscess	1
Adult Subdural Empyema	15
Adult Cranial Extradural Abscess	21
Adult Cranial Fungal and Parasitic Infections	25
References	28

Adult Cerebral Abscess

Clinical Scenarios

For paediatric cerebral abscess, cranial extradural abscess, and subdural empyema see paediatric section of the book (Varthalitis, El-Adwan and Usher, *Child with an Acute Intracranial Infection*, Elements in Emergency Neurosurgery, Cambridge University Press, forthcoming).

A fifty-five-year-old lady presented with a few weeks of feeling unwell and was found unconscious at home. She was initially GCS 15, then became more confused and agitated. CT with contrast of the head showed left middle ear opacity and an intracerebral abscess within the left temporal lobe. She underwent a neuro-navigated burr hole drainage of left temporal abscess and a left-sided modified radical mastoidectomy by our ENT colleagues. She initially recovered well and was on long-term antibiotics (meropenem and metronidazole). However, a month after her initial surgery, her abscess recurred despite being on antibiotics. Another neuro-navigated aspiration was performed. This time the abscess was successfully treated and follow-up imaging only showed a small area of enhancement within the abscess wall, likely representing the remnant abscess capsule (Figure 1).

Core Knowledge

Definition

Adult cerebral abscess (CA) is a focal infection of the brain that begins as a localised area of cerebritis that eventually progresses into a collection of pus within the brain.

Epidemiology

It has an incidence of 0.4/100,000 per year (1) in the developed world, but it is found to be higher in developing countries. It has a female preponderance (M:F, 1:3) and represents around 1% of all radiologically diagnosed intracranial space-occupying lesions.

Aetiology

The microorganism that causes CA can arrive to the brain via three different routes. The most common is haematogenous spread from infections arising from sites such as the heart (acute bacterial endocarditis), lungs (lower respiratory chest infections, lung abscess, and empyema), skin (cellulitis), tooth extraction, bone (osteomyelitis), or bowel. Contiguous spread occurs from sites adjacent to the brain, such as infective sinusitis and tooth infections.

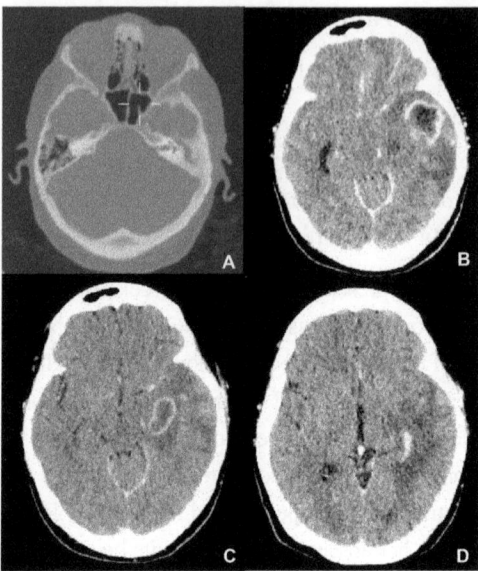

Figure 1 Clinical scenario for adult cerebral abscess
(A) CT head on bone windows showing left mastoid air cell opacification.
(B) Initial CT with contrast showing a ring-enhancing lesion in the left temporal lobe. This was treated via a neuro-navigated aspiration of the abscess.
(C) One month following the initial treatment a follow-up scan showed that there was a recurrence of the abscess.
(D) Three months from the initial scan, almost complete resolution of the abscess is seen with a small area of enhancement.

Infections of the air sinuses can lead to local osteomyelitis and spread to the brain via emissary vein phlebitis. In contiguous abscesses, the location of the sinusitis is adjacent to the location of the CA. For example, middle ear infections and mastoid air sinusitis tend to cause temporal or cerebellar abscess, whereas sphenoid sinusitis tends to cause cavernous sinus thrombosis and temporal lobe abscesses. Tooth infections tend to cause frontal lobe abscesses via contiguous spread through calvarial osteomyelitis or can occur within four weeks of a dental procedure through haematological spread (2). The third route for infection to spread to the brain is through direct inoculation, either from neurosurgical procedures or from penetrating head injury. Cerebral abscess has been described in a variety of neurosurgical procedures, including craniotomies and/or implantation of intracranial devices. The causative organisms in penetrating head injury can be from the air sinuses if they are along the projectiles path or from normal flora from the skin or clothes (Figure 2).

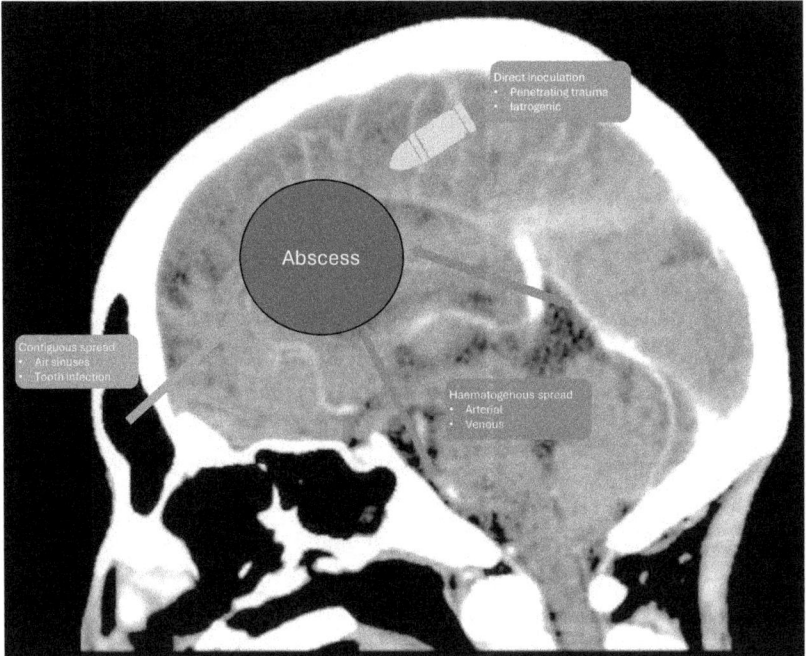

Figure 2 Infective routes for cerebral abscesses

Risk Factors

Patients who are immunocompromised or have pulmonary shunting, in the form of congenital heart disease or conditions such as Osler–Weber–Rendu syndrome, are at a higher risk of CA. Immunosuppression can be from AIDS or medical treatment such as chemotherapy or long-term steroids use. Five per cent of patients with Osler–Weber–Rendu syndrome developed CA secondary to the pulmonary arteriovenous fistula that causes pulmonary shunting (3).

Pathogen

A study by Helweg-Larsen et al. in 2012 has shown that the most common pathogens found within CA were Streptococci (54%), Staphylococci (15%), Gram-negative bacteria (8%), anaerobic bacteria (17%), and Nocardia (2%) (1). The incidence of no growth in pus cultures obtained from drainage of the CA can be as high as 41% (4). This is likely to be due to the use of antibiotics prior to abscess drainage. The type of pathogens is closely associated with the source of infection, for example, strep. Milleri and strep. Anginosus are commonly seen in abscess due to frontal and ethmoidal sinusitis, whereas staph. Aureus and Clostridium spp. are seen in direct inoculation from penetrating brain injuries

(5). Cerebral abscess associated with lung abscesses can be due to Fusobacterium, actinomyces, and Nocardia Spp. Fusobacterium, actinomyces are commonly seen in CA secondary to dental infections (6). Pathogens such as Mycobacterium, toxoplasma Gondii, Nocardia asteroids, listeria monocytogenes, and fungal infections (Aspergillus fumitagus and Cryptococcus Neoformans) are found in immunocompromised patients with CA (7).

Stages of Abscess Formation

Britt et al. using a canine model of infection with α-haemolytic streptococci defined four different stages of in the formation of a CA (8). Although these stages are not distinct, they are a good model of understanding how abscesses form and how they transform radiologically over time (Table 1). The four stages are early cerebritis, late cerebritis, early capsule formation, and late capsule formation.

Early cerebritis occurs between days 1 and 3. The core of the infective elements contains acute inflammatory cells with bacteria present on gram staining. The border of the involved brain and infective element contains acute inflammatory cells. During this period, a collagenous capsule made of reticulin starts to form. The surrounding brain starts to show marked oedema. Radiologically during the early cerebritis stage, there is partial ring enhancement on CT with contrast, but later this ring enhancement gets more pronounced. Steroids given during the early cerebritis stage can dampen down the degree of contrast enhancement. Late cerebritis starts around day 4 and ends around day 10. During this time, the core of the infective elements starts to become necrotic and enlarges to its maximum size. The previously acute inflammatory cell border will now have macrophages and fibroblasts. Due to the presence of the fibroblasts, there is now a rapid formation of the collagenous wall. The surrounding brain oedema is still present with appearance of reactive astrocytes within the normal brain. During the first two cerebritis stages, the T1-weighted and T2-weighted MRI show hypointensity and hyperintensity of the affected brain, respectively. During this period there is a delay in diffusion of contrast into the lucent centre, whereas later in the capsule formation stages, there is less diffusion of contrast material into the lucent centre.

In the early capsule formation stage, which begins and ends from day 10 and day 13, respectively, there is a start in the decrease in the volume of the necrotic centre. There is also a further increase in fibroblast and macrophage translocation into the inflammatory border. There is also now maximal neovascularization of the abscess. The collagen within the capsule is maturing. One of the characteristic features of the early capsule formation stage is regression of

Table 1 Stages of cerebral abscess formation. (References: Britt et al. (8) and Erdogan and Cansever (2008))

	Early cerebritis	Late cerebritis	Early capsule formation	Late capsule formation
Days	1–3	4–9	10–13	> 14
Resistance of capsule to needle aspiration	Intermediate resistance	No resistance	No resistance	Firm resistance. Has 'give' on entering
Necrotic centre	Acute inflammatory cells; bacteria present on gram stain	Enlarging necrotic centre reaching maximal size	Decrease in necrotic centre	Further decrease in necrotic centre
Inflammatory border	Acute inflammatory cells	Inflammatory cells, macrophages, and fibroblast	Increasing numbers of fibroblast and macrophages	Further increase in number of fibroblasts
Cerebritis and neovascularity	Rapid perivascular infiltration of neutrophils, plasma cells, and mononuclear cells	Maximal extent of cerebritis Rapid increase in new vessel formation	Maximal degree of neovascularization	Cerebritis restricted to the outside of the collagen capsule. Reduced neovascularity
Collagenous capsule	Reticulin formation begins by day 3	Appearance of fibroblasts with rapid formation of reticulin	Evolution of mature collagen	Capsule completed by end of second week
Reactive gliosis and cerebral oedema	Marked cerebral oedema	Prominent cerebral oedema Appearance of reactive astrocytes	Regression of cerebral oedema Increase in reactive astrocytes	Regression of cerebral oedema. Marked gliosis outside capsule by 3rd week

Table 1 (cont.)

	Early cerebritis	Late cerebritis	Early capsule formation	Late capsule formation
CT	Partial ring contrast enhancement on day 1 evolving to well-developed ring enhancement by day 3. Steroids reduce degree of contrast enhancement (especially in cerebritis)	Thick ring enhancement. Diffusion of contrast medium into the lucent centre on delayed scans (30–60 minutes after contrast infusion) is salient CT finding of cerebritis stage	Ring enhancement with less diffusion of contrast material into the lucent centre	Ring enhancement without diffusion of contrast material into the lucent centre

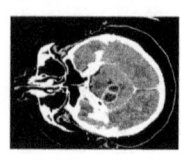
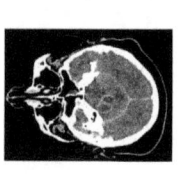
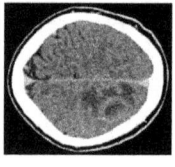

MRI

T1:
Hypointense
T2:
Hyperintense

T1:
Core → hypointense,
Capsule → mildly hyperintense
Perilesional oedema → hypointense

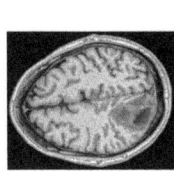

T2:
Core → iso/hyperintense
Capsule → hypointense
Perilesional oedema → hyperintense
DWI:
Restricted:

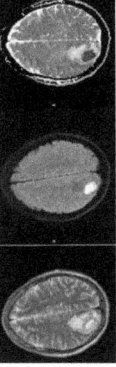

Table 1 (cont.)

Early cerebritis	Late cerebritis	Early capsule formation	Late capsule formation
		T1+C: Ring-enhancing lesion 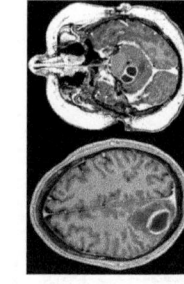	

cerebral oedema. In the late capsule formation stage, which occurs after day 14, the cerebritis is restricted to the outside of the now matured collagen capsule. Due to the presence of a matured collagen capsule, this is the stage where one would feel a firm resistance when passing a needle into the abscess. The capsule facing the cortical surface has higher oxygen availability and thus can form a thicker capsular wall when compared to the capsular wall facing the deeper ventricular surface. This explains why CA tends to rupture into the ventricular system rather than rupturing on the cortical surface. The surrounding brain will start to show signs of gliosis. Radiologically on MRI the necrotic core will be hypointense on T1-weighted sequences, and hyper or iso intense on T2-weighted sequences. This is in contrast to the capsule, which is hyperintense on T1-weighted imaging and hypointense on T2-weighted imaging. Diffusion-weighted imaging (DWI) will show restriction due to the presence of pus. T1 post-contrast studies will show the classical ring-enhancing lesion.

Clinical Presentation

Patients with CA frequently present with headache, fever (60%), nausea or vomiting (40%), and/or focal neurological (57%) deficits depending on the location of the abscess (1). Frontal lobe abscess is more common than temporal or parietal abscess. Later during the disease, the patient can also present with seizure (21%) and impaired consciousness (45%). These symptoms are due to the mass effect and local irritatory effects of the perilesional oedema and the CA itself. Unlike other intracranial infections, CA does not generally present with meningism. Sudden worsening of the headache, accompanied by the new onset of meningism, may suggest the rupture of the abscess into the ventricular space (9).

Investigation

White cell count and CRP can be raised or normal in patients with CA. Blood cultures should be done if patients are pyrexial. Lumbar puncture should be avoided as there is a risk of herniation if the CA is large enough to cause a significant mass effect. It is important to be aware that normal inflammatory markers do not rule out a CA.

Samples obtained from the abscess by surgical drainage can be studied through gram staining and microscopy for can help guide immediate antibiotic choice. Abscess culture can allow identification of the pathogen involved and also allow for antibiotic sensitivity testing.

Radiologically the classical description of CA is of a ring-enhancing lesion. Cerebral abscess tends to localise in the grey-white matter junction and in watershed areas of the brain where the oxygen tension is lower. They tend to be multiple in 21% of cases (1). CT with contrast shows a uniform thickness ring-enhancing lesion with surrounding cerebral hypodensity signifying cerebral oedema.

MRI is more sensitive than CT in detecting CA. It can detect early cerebritis and satellite lesions that tend to be missed on CT. T1-weighted imaging shows the central necrotic core that is low intensity surrounded by a slightly hyper-intense rim representing the capsule. Surrounding the capsule, the surrounding vasogenic oedema in the brain will be low intensity. T2-weighted or FLAIR imaging shows that the rim is of low intensity whereas the area of cerebral oedema is high intensity. T1-weighted post-contrast imaging shows a ring-enhancing lesion.

In immunocompromised patients, there may be a relative lack of contrast enhancement which can make diagnosis difficult. Due to the presence of necrotic material within the abscess core which can restrict the motion of water, there is a high signal intensity on DWI and low apparent apparent diffusion coefficient (ADC) values within the core of the cavity. DWI can be used to monitor treatment response, and it is most useful in differentiating between a neoplastic process vs an infectious one (Table 2) (10).

MRS shows elevated peaks of metabolites that are associated with hypoxia and cellular breakdown, such as lipids/lactate, succinate, acetate, and amino acids (alanine, valine, leucine, and isoleucine). MRS can also help differentiate the various types of CA: Pyogenic abscesses have raised cytosolic amino acids, acetate, and succinate; Tubercular abscesses have raised lipid/lactate peaks; and fungal abscesses showed raised lipid, lactate, amino acids, and trehalose peaks (11). Like DWI MRS can help delineate infection from tumour (Table 2).

Acute Management

The goal of CA treatment is to obtain a sample for diagnosis, reduce the infective load within the brain, and relieve the pressure effects of the abscess onto the brain. The mainstay of treatment is surgical aspiration or excision of the abscess followed by long-term antibiotics. The primary source of infection should also be treated acutely. This can be done with the assistance of ENT or maxillofacial surgery. It is reasonable to give anti-convulsants prophylactically in some cases, but must be started if there is evidence of seizure activity, with Levetiracetam the most used initial agent. If seizures are not well controlled with a single agent, another agent can be added with neurology advice.

Steroids use in the context of CA have been controversial. The theory behind their use is that it can improve the vasogenic oedema help control mass effect.

However, steroids can decrease host immunity, delay the formation of an abscess wall therefore allowing more destruction of the surrounding normal brain. Studies have shown that steroid use has been associated with higher mortality, and it does not seem to improve overall outcomes (1). If they are going to be used to control mass effect, this should be for a short duration.

Pure antibiotic treatment of a CA without surgery is used in certain clinical circumstances. One would be the late referral of a patient that was showing signs of improvement after starting antibiotics, if the lesion were small (<1.7 cm), or if the patient had an irreversible coagulopathy. Local anaesthetic drainage can be considered in patients with medical comorbidity. Patients with multiple small abscesses or the abscess in a poorly accessible location (12) can be treated with antibiotics alone and this is often done in the paediatric population with associated congenital heart disease/endocarditis where the organism is known.

Pure antibiotic treatment is less effective in the treatment of CA because the pathogens are contained within a thick capsular wall with poor blood supply, and the acidic environment within the abscess readily denatures the antibiotics. The choice of antibiotic agents should be discussed with the local infectious diseases team. The choice of antibiotics is based on the source of infection, which dictates the type of pathogen involved. For infections from sinusitis or tooth infections, a 3rd-generation cephalosporin and metronidazole should be used, whereas for infections from a post-traumatic or post-surgical source a 3rd-generation cephalosporin and vancomycin should be used. The duration of antibiotic should be for at least six to eight weeks, and this should be guided by clinical, biochemical, and radiographic response to treatment (12).

Indications for surgical management of CA are if the abscess is expanding towards the ventricles, neurological deterioration, failure of pure antibiotic treatment, uncertainty of diagnosis, raised ICP and mass effect, presence of a foreign body within the abscess, abscesses that are large (>2.5 cm) and/or multiloculated (13). The surgical options are needle aspiration, open surgical drainage, or surgical excision. Needle aspiration is the easiest to do with the lowest complication rate. It can be done for most patients and can be done under General or local anaesthetic with a scalp block. It is also the technique of choice for deeply seated lesions. One of the downsides of needle aspiration is that it does not allow complete removal of the infective material, therefore resulting in a higher recurrence of the abscess. Open surgical drainage, on the other hand, may reduce recurrence risk and on occasions has been shown to reduce antibiotic duration (1). It can allow for any foreign body to be removed and to drain any multiloculated lesions. However, this procedure is more complicated and has a higher complication rate than needle aspiration. Surgical drainage should only be performed in abscesses that are in the late capsular phase, where there is well formed collagenous capsular wall. Surgical

Table 2 Differentiating intracranial tumour vs abscess. (References : Cartes-Zumelzu et al. (10) and Luthra et al. (11)).

Features	Tumour	Abscess
CT/MRI	Less uniform ring-enhancing thickness	More uniform ring-enhancing thickness
	Relatively less oedema	Relatively more oedema
	Relatively slower growing	Relatively faster growing
DWI	Core DWI hypointense, high ADC values	Core DWI hyperintense, low ADC values
	Wall DWI hyperintense, low ADC values	Wall DWI hypointense, high ADC values
MRS	Decrease in NAA and creatine peaks	Decrease/absent in NAA and Cr peaks
	Increase in choline, lipids, and lactate peaks.	Increase in lipids/lactate, succinate, acetate, and amino acids (alanine, valine, leucine, and isoleucine) peaks

excision like surgical drainage can only be done during the late capsular stage but unlike surgical drainage here the abscess is removed like a tumour. As a result of this surgical excision has a higher risk of damaging the viable brain surrounding the abscess. Surgical excision is usually only employed for abscesses that contain a foreign body, known fungal or nocardia abscesses or needle drainage-resistant abscesses. If there are multiple abscesses, the largest lesion or the most symptomatic abscess should be targeted in the first instance (14).

Technical Note – For Needle Aspiration of CA

Preoperatively measure the volume of CA on available imaging. This can be done using your local Picture Archiving and Communication System (PACS) or the ABC/2 formula, where A, B, and C are the largest length of the CA in all three dimensions that are at right angles to each other. A needle aspiration is an image-guided minimally invasive approach that can be done with frame or frameless stereotaxis and/or ultrasound guidance. The author's preference is with frameless stereotaxis using Neuronavigation for deep CA and USS guidance as backup or for more superficial CA. Plan a trajectory with the shortest route, not traversing any major vessel or ventricles, and preferably choose a gyrus rather than a sulcus as the entry point. The target of the aspiration needle should stay away from the deepest, ventricular-facing wall so to prevent accidental fenestration of the CA into the ventricle. The frameless stereotactic apparatus should be set up according to the manufacturer's guidelines. The hair is clipped, and a small incision is made as to allow a perforator to be used to make a burr hole. The burr hole is made so that the needle is located at the centre of the burr hole. The burr hole sometimes needs to be bevelled to ensure that the aspiration needle is not touching the surrounding bone. A 15-blade stab incision is made on the dura. A bipolar diathermy is then passed through this dural defect, and the cortex is coagulated. This ensures that the dura is only opened slightly to prevent CSF loss and brain shift, and at the same time to perform a corticortomy. The frameless stereotactic apparatus is then repositioned into place and the needle is passed smoothly without obstructions into the CA. Often, when penetrating through the abscess capsule, some resistance can be felt. Aspirate the contents of the CA until dry and send the sample for both microbiology and pathology analysis. Measure the volume of CA aspirated before removing the needle and closing.

If an ultrasound is used instead, the authors prefer using the small probe with a probe guide. The entry point should be planned on CT and the entry point marked out using callipers. A perforator is used to perform a burr hole that is then widened to allow access for both the aspiration needle and the ultrasound probe. The durotomy and corticortomy is performed as previously discussed. At the end of the aspiration, the USS can be used to visualise any remaining large collections.

Management Algorithms

See cerebral abscess flow diagram (Figure 3)

PITFALLS AND PEARLS

- LP is generally non-diagnostic for CA and can be dangerous in the context of raised intracranial pressure.
- Steroids should only be used for short duration, usage of more than a few days can worsen outcomes.
- Early diagnosis and treatment to prevent the progression of CA is key.
- MRI is the most useful diagnostic and monitoring modality. It can be useful if differentiating tumours from CA.
- Be wary of abscesses that are adjacent to the ventricle as rupture of an abscess into a ventricle has high morbidity and mortality.

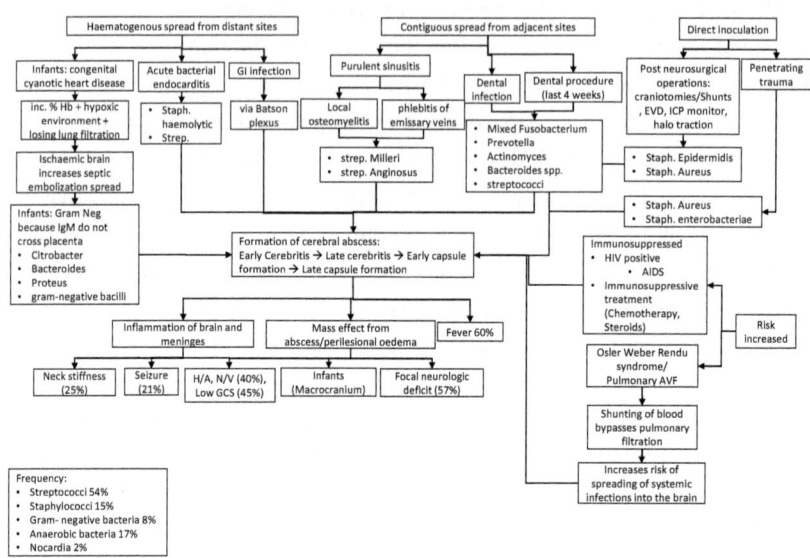

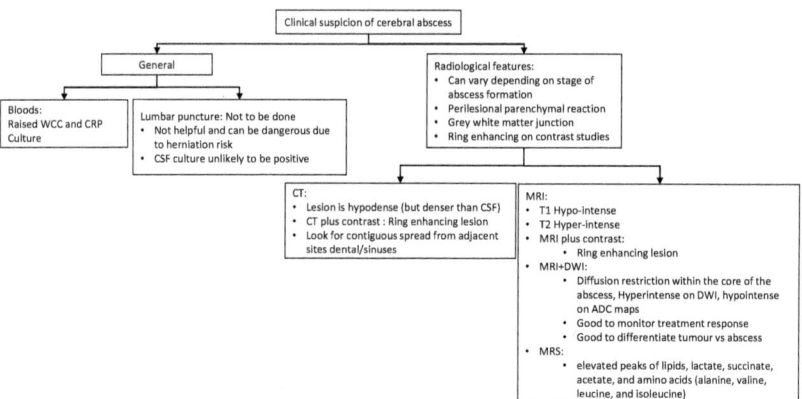

Figure 3 Cerebral abscess pathophysiology, investigations, and management

Intracranial Abscess in Adults

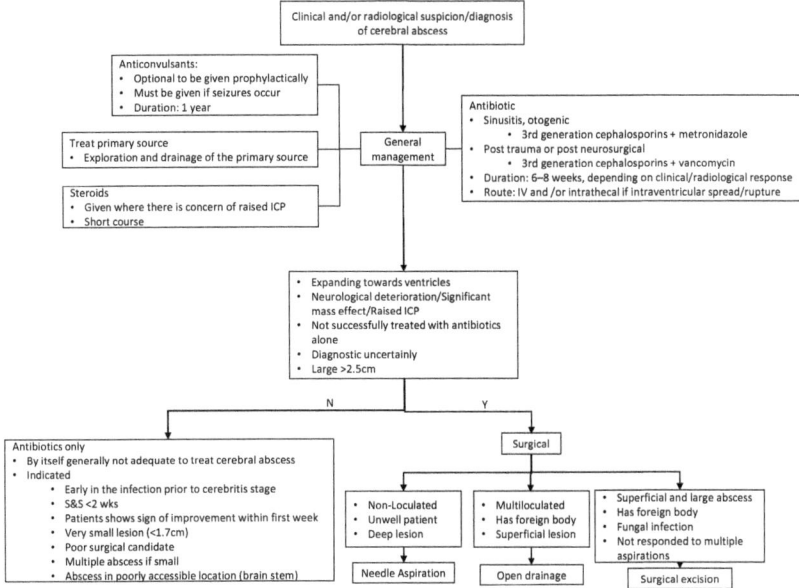

Figure 3 (cont.)

Adult Subdural Empyema

Clinical Scenarios

A twenty-year-old male patient presented with two weeks of feeling unwell with nasal discharge and fevers. Patient had difficulty opening his eyes and a frontal headache and forehead swelling. CT with contrast showed an enhancing subdural collection and opacification of the maxillary and ethmoidal sinuses. This was treated via a left frontal craniotomy and endoscopic sinus surgery. The patient was placed on long-term antibiotics and the three-month follow-up scan showed only residual reactive enhancement of the dura (Figure 4).

Core Knowledge

Definition

Adult subdural empyema (SE) is a collection of pus in the subdural space.

Epidemiology

It occurs more often in males (M:F, 3:1), peaking in the third decade of life. It is five times less common than CAs (15).

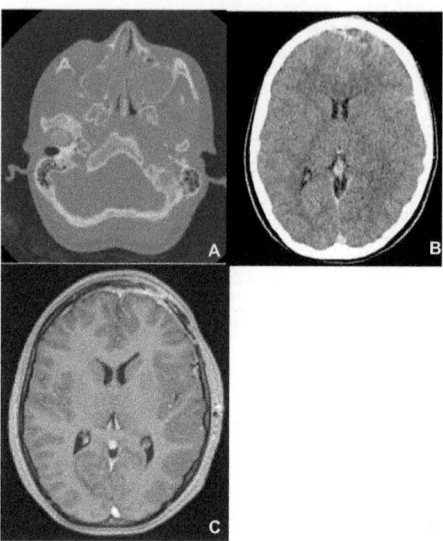

Figure 4 Clinical scenario for adult cerebral subdural empyema
(A) CT head on bone windows showing maxillary and ethmoidal sinuses opacification.
(B) Initial CT with contrast showing an extradural collection. This was treated via a craniotomy and endoscopic sinus surgery.
(C) Three months following the initial treatment a follow-up MRI scan with contrast showed that there is only residual reactive enhancement of the dura.

Aetiology

Similar to a CA, the causative microorganism can reach the brain haematogenously, by contiguous spread or by direct inoculation. In contrast to an abscess, the haematogenous route is less common and most arise from contiguous spread from infected air sinuses or by direct inoculation from neurosurgical procedures or penetrating brain injuries. The most common surgical procedure associated with SE is drainage of chronic subdural haematomas (CSDH). This is especially true when subdural haematomas are drained via a craniotomy rather than burr holes (16).

Pathogen

The most common causative pathogens are aerobic and anaerobic streptococci, which are associated with infections of the middle ear. Post craniotomy, the commonest organisms are staphylococci and gram-negative species, whereas Propionibacterium acnes, a ubiquitous skin commensal is commonly found in CSDH patients (17). Staphylococci and gram-negative species infections are also found in patients with penetrating head injuries. Failure to identify an organism

Table 3 Microbiological incidence of subdural empyema https://doctorlib.info/infectiology/infections-central-nervous-system/34.html Infections of the Central Nervous System, 4th Ed.

Organism	Incidence
Aerobic streptococci	36%
Anaerobic streptococci	10%
Coagulase-positive staphylococci	9%
Coagulase-negative staphylococci	3%
Aerobic gram-negative bacilli	10%
Other anaerobes	6%
Culture negative studies	29%

can occur in up to 40% of cases, and this may be due to previous exposure to antibiotics and difficulties in culturing anaerobic organisms (Table 3).

Pathology

SE has the propensity to spread rapidly due to a lack of a fibrin capsule and anatomical barriers in the subdural space. Most (80%) SE are localised over the convexity, but some do localise in the para-falcine region (20%). Concomitant presentation of a CA or an epidural abscess occurs in up to 22% and 17% of cases, respectively.

Clinical Presentation

In contrast to patients with CA, who frequently present with headache (86%) and fever (95%), in SE patients 83% present with meningism and 80% with unilateral hemispheric dysfunction. Affected patients can deteriorate rapidly with seizures in 63% and reduced conscious level in 76% (18). The median time from the onset of symptoms to diagnosis is two days (19). Other common symptoms include tenderness over the affected air sinuses (42%) and forehead or eye swelling secondary to emissary vein thrombosis may occur (20). The clinical presentation is secondary to the mass effect, inflammation of the brain and meninges and thrombophlebitis of the cerebral veins or venous sinuses.

Investigation

White cell count and CRP can be raised in affected patients. Blood cultures should be done if the patient is pyrexial. Lumbar puncture should be avoided as there is a risk of herniation, and the yield of a positive culture is low unless there is an associated meningitis.

The radiological features of a SE a crescent-shaped collection with dense enhancement of the medial membrane (21). As it is in the subdural space, it will not be constrained by suture lines and overlies the surface of the brain.

On a plain CT scan, it is a hypodense collection that is hard to differentiate from a chronic subdural haematoma, and small lesions may be difficult to see. In a contrast-enhanced CT, a brightly enhancing rim is suggestive of an empyema but a lack of contrast enhancement does not fully exclude a SE, as it could mean that the empyema is chronic and is well organised (16).

On MRI, T1-weighted sequences show a hypointense and T2-weighted sequences show a hyperintense subdural collection. Contrast-enhanced T1-weighted MRI is more sensitive than CT with contrast in detecting SEs. It is also useful for identifying collections located at the skull base, post fossa and along the falx cerebri. Subdural empyema restricts on DWI. It can help distinguish SE from subdural haematoma (22).

Acute Management

Almost all SEs need surgical drainage due to poor antibiotic penetration into the subdural space. Pure antibiotic management can be trialled for patients with no neurological deficit, small collections and patients that have had an early good symptomatic response (23). Delayed treatment for more than seventy-two hours is associated with a poorer outcome. Antibiotic treatment should ideally be started after surgical sampling of the subdural has occurred. However, broad-based empirical antibiotic therapy should not be delayed in a septic, systemically unwell patient. The choice of antibiotic should be targeted on the presumed source of the infection. After obtaining culture and sensitivity results, the antibiotics should be modified as per microbiology advice. Duration of antibiotics should be at least six weeks and guided by clinical, biochemical, and radiological responses (24).

Like CA prophylactic antiepileptic medication should be considered but anticonvulsants must be started if there is any evidence of seizure secondary to the SE. The primary source of the infection should also be treated or drained as soon as possible to prevent recurrence of the SE.

Subdural empyema can be drained via a burr hole, craniotomy, or a craniectomy. Burr hole drainage is suitable for an empyema that is not viscous or loculated. Since it is a simpler operation, it is suitable for critically unwell patients. However, burr hole drainage has a higher recurrence rate, and about 20% of cases will require a craniotomy for more definitive treatment. The use of a craniotomy is generally indicated for thick organised empyema (16). It is also more effective in treating loculated empyema. Generally, a wide craniotomy is needed. Frequently, there is an organised membrane on the surface of the cortex, and if this is not flushable with normal saline washes, they should not be stripped from the brain, as this can lead to cortical injury and bleeding. A craniectomy is sometimes needed if there is a worry about brain swelling underlying the empyema. This is especially true, the SE has started to affect the cortex and cause cerebritis. A craniectomy is also sometimes required if the bone overlying the empyema is infected and de-vascularized in the context of a post-operative or post-penetrative traumatic head injury. All three methods have been shown to be effective if empyema can be successfully drained (25). Early post-operative imaging will confirm the effectiveness of drainage and will guide further surgical management.

Technical Note – Craniotomy for SE

Preoperatively study the MRI and/or CT scan to identify the location of the SE and if there are any interhemispheric/skull base components of it. Plan a craniotomy centred around the SE. Skin incision made, and a bone flap is raised. The dura is then opened. Pus collected and sent for microbiology analysis. Wash pus out with warm saline. Do not attempt to peel any pus that is adherent to the cortex. Wash out any pus in the skull base or interhemispheric space, but be careful not to over-flush these spaces with wash and keep these spaces open with long-patties to prevent the brain from swelling above the craniotomy site. Clean the dura. Agents like Hydrogen Peroxide can be used, but be aware that they can foam and cause brain expansion if there is it is trapped in tight spaces within the brain. Standard closure should then be done. Frequently, if there is a concomitant infective source, we would invite the ENT surgeon or the Maxillofacial surgeon to drain the primary infective source.

Management Algorithms

See subdural empyema flow diagram (Figure 5).

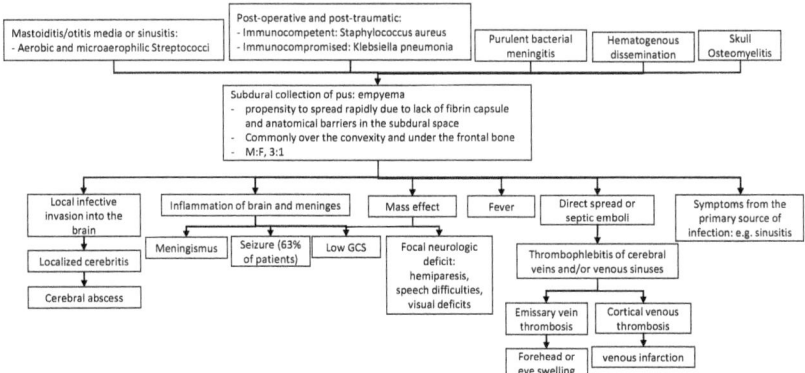

Figure 5 Subdural empyema pathophysiology, investigations, and management

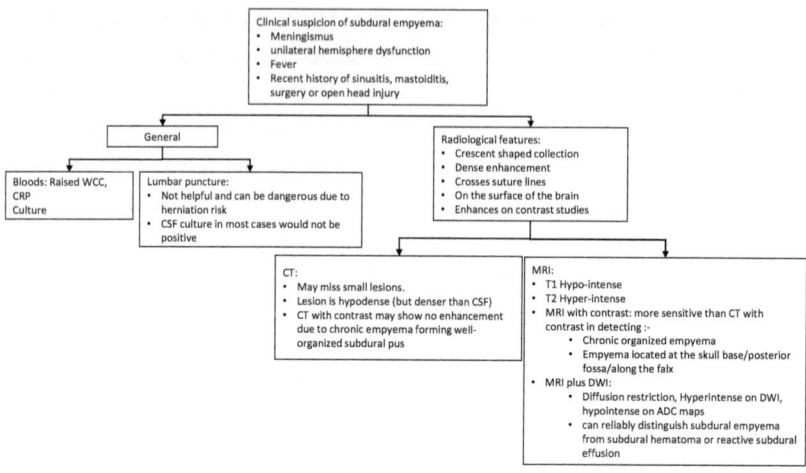
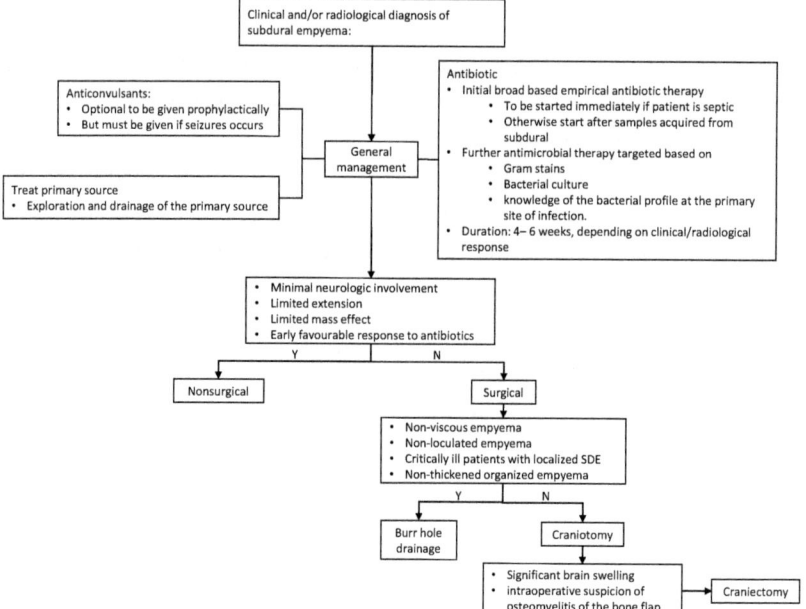

Figure 5 (cont.)

> PITFALLS AND PEARLS
>
> - An LP is generally non-diagnostic for SE and can be dangerous in the context of raised intracranial pressure due to mass effect.
> - MRI can be useful in differentiating SE from subdural haematomas.
> - Although tempting, do not attempt to peel off any adherent membranes from the surface of the brain, as this can cause harm to the patient.

Adult Cranial Extradural Abscess

Clinical Scenarios

An eighteen-year-old female presented with fever, headache, and nasal discharge. CT with contrast showed opacification of the Maxillary sinus and an extradural enhancing collection. She underwent a right frontal brainlab-guided drainage of extradural abscess and an endoscopic sinus surgery. As the burr hole is over the forehead, we used Hydrocet a bone cement to cover the defect. (Figure 6)

Core Knowledge

Definition

Adult cranial extradural abscess (CEA) is a collection of pus that arises between the skull and the dura.

Epidemiology

It is less common than CA and SE. It affects all ages and represents 1.8% of all intracranial infections (26).

Aetiology

Cranial extradural abscess commonly occurs by contiguous spread from sinusitis or mastoiditis. Other sources of contiguous spread are skull osteomyelitis or dental infections. Direct spread through neurosurgical procedures or open skull fractures can also occur.

Pathogen

The microorganisms associated with CEA are similar to the spectrum seen in SE, such as Staph Aureus, Streptococci, and gram-negative bacilli (27).

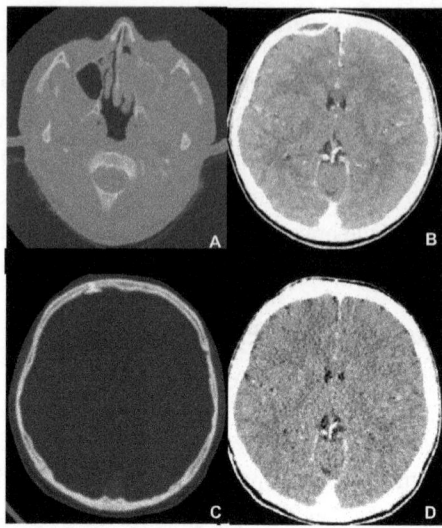

Figure 6 Clinical scenario for adult extradural abscess
(A) CT head on bone windows showing left maxillary sinus opacification.
(B) Initial CT with contrast showing an enhancing extradural collection under the right frontal bone. This was treated via a burr hole aspiration of the collection.
(C) CT on bone window at one month following the initial treatment showing that the burr hole was covered by Hydrocet, a bone cement.
(D) CT with contrast at one month from the initial scan, shows complete resolution of the abscess.

Pathology

The growing inflammatory mass of the CEA slowly dissects the dura away from the skull, which explains the insidious onset of clinical presentation. Most CEA are on the convexity and rarely occur in the skull base as the dura is more tightly adherent to the skull.

Clinical Presentation

Patients with CEA frequently present with fever (57%), headache (37%), and meningism (35%). A frontal subperiosteal abscess, also known as 'Pott's puffy tumour', can be associated with a contiguous frontal CEA (46%) will present with forehead swelling. If there are associated seizures (11%) present, it might suggest meningitis or cerebral involvement (26). In CEA secondary to a neurosurgical cause, wound infection is almost always present (95.7%). Complications that can arise from CEA are skull osteomyelitis and thrombosis of emissary veins.

Investigation

Similar to CA and SE, lumbar puncture should be avoided as there is a risk of herniation and a low yield of a positive CSF microbiology result (26).

Radiologically CEA is described as a lentiform-shaped enhancing collection. CT might show bony destruction or mastoid opacification. MRI is useful to detect small abscesses and abscesses around the skull based that are easily missed on CT (28). Diffusion-weighted MRI can help differentiate SE from CEAs. High signal intensity on DWI tends to favour a SE diagnosis, while for CEA, a low or mix signal intensity is more frequently seen (29). Diffusion weighted MRI can also help differentiate whether a post op extradural collection is a sterile or infective.

Acute Management

Management of CEA consists of drainage of the abscess, controlling the source of the infection and antibiotics. Empirical antibiotics should be started immediately after microbiological samples have been taken or if the patient is septic. For spontaneous CEA, a 3rd-generation cephalosporin and metronidazole should be given, while for post-operative or post-traumatic CEA, vancomycin and meropenem should be used instead. After obtaining culture results, antibiotic therapy should be modified according to the sensitivities.

The aim of surgery is to reduce the mass effect of the CEA, reduce the infective load and obtain material for culture. In contrast to SE, a more limited surgical procedure in the form of a burr hole/craniectomy to allow adequate drainage of the extradural space is usually employed. A craniectomy is sometimes needed to resect localised osteomyelitis. It is also important to drain/treat any contiguous pathology at the same time as draining the cranial collection.

Management Algorithms

See extradural abscess flow diagram (Figure 7).

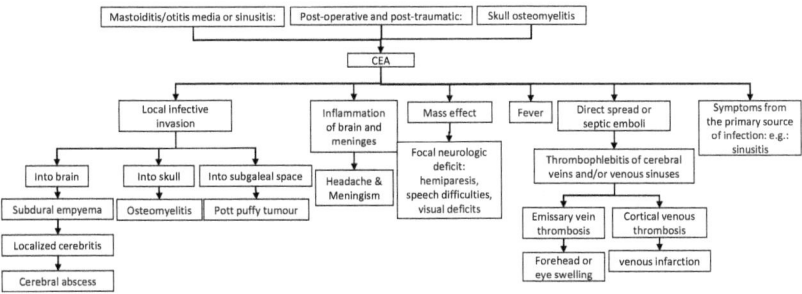

Figure 7 Extradural abscess pathophysiology, investigations, and management

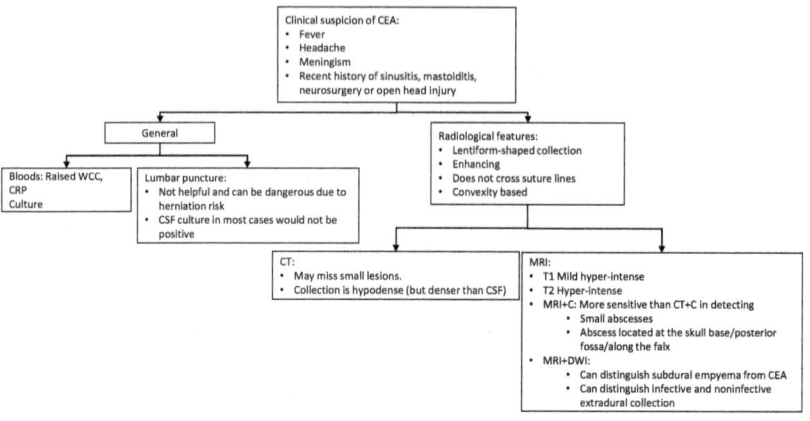

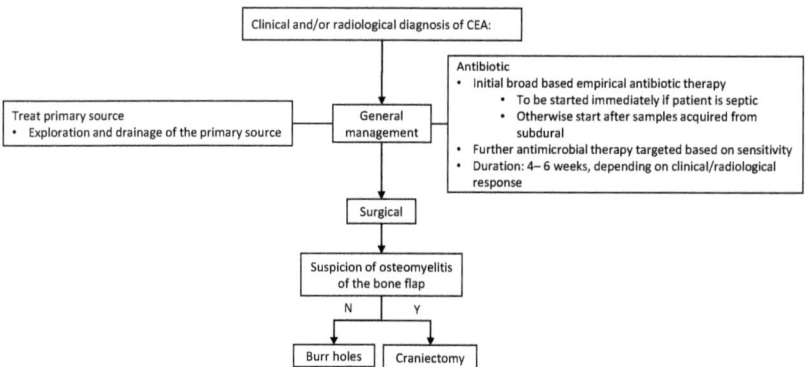

Figure 7 (cont.)

PITFALLS AND PEARLS

- LP is non-diagnostic for CEA and can be dangerous in the context of raised intracranial pressure.
- DWI sequences are useful in differentiating CEA from SE and sterile from infective post-operative infective extradural collections.
- CEA has a sharp demarcation, slower progression rate, and an indolent course when compared to subdural collection.
- Infected bone should be removed via a craniectomy.

Adult Cranial Fungal and Parasitic Infections

Most fungal and parasitic infections of the CNS are managed medically. In this section, we will describe three fungal and parasitical infections that may require surgical intervention. These are Cryptococcosis, Cysticercosis, and Echinococcus. For paediatric cranial fungal and parasitic infections, see paediatric section of the Element.

Cryptococcosis

Cryptococcosis is the second most common cerebral fungal infection, with the first being candidiasis. It is due to cryptococcosis neoformans, which is normally found in bird faeces. It can present in two forms, the more common cryptococcal meningitis and the rarer crytococcoma, also known as mucinous pseudocyst. Cryptococcal meningitis occurs more frequently in patients who are immunocompromised (30). It can present as fever, tiredness, headaches, and with signs of meningeal irritation. The organism gains access to the human body through inhalation of basidiospores, which then spread to the brain via the haemato-lymphatic route. Some patients can present with raised intracranial pressure. Radiologically, there can be dilatation of the Virchow–Robbins spaces. Cryptococcoma is exclusively found in patients with AIDS with the lesions arising in the basal ganglia. The diagnosis of cryptococcosis is established via positivity in the serum or CSF cryptococcus antigen. It is treated with Amphotericin B and fluconazole for two to six weeks, depending on CSF clearance of the antigen (31). Raised intracranial pressure may need to be managed with daily lumbar punctures, a lumbar drain or CSF shunting.

Cysticercosis

Cysticercosis is the most common CNS parasitic infection. It is due to Taenia Solium, which is a tapeworm where the human body is the definitive host. Taenia Solium, if it infects a human in its adult phase of life, causes taeniasis, however if it infects a human in its larval form, it causes cysticercosis. Humans can ingest the eggs via contaminated food or water. In the duodenum, the eggs hatch and burrow through the intestinal wall to enter the lymphatic or vascular system. The newly hatched embryos, also known as oncospheres, enter the brain where it forms a cyst which eventually present as Neurocysticercosis (32).

Neurocysticercosis occurs in 60–92% of cases of cysticercosis (33). It can take up to two to five years from the ingestion of eggs to symptomatic neurocysticercosis. Cysts are commonly found in the subarachnoid spaces or within the brain parenchyma. Rarely, it can also be found within the ventricular system. These cysts can cause local inflammation in the form of vasculitis, leading to stroke, meningitis, arachnoiditis, or ependymitis or obstruction leading to hydrocephalus. Most patients present with seizures (69%), headaches (46%), and/or visual disturbance (13%). The diagnosis is made based on radiological studies and serological testing. Eosinophils in the blood and CSF can be raised. Enzyme-linked immunoelectrotransfer blot against anti-cysticercal antibodies has a high sensitivity and specificity (34). Radiologically, a cystic lesion with an associated scolex, which is seen as a 1- to 3-mm mural nodule is diagnostic.

Many cysts resolve spontaneously therefore the use of Anthelmintics such as Praziquantel and Albendazole is not necessarily needed (35). These drugs, although have been shown to increase the likelihood of radiologic cyst resolution, they do carry significant side effects such as headaches, dizziness, and seizures. Generally, Seizures secondary to neurocysticercosis respond well to a single antiepileptic agent (36). The most used antiepileptic agents are phenytoin and carbamazepine. Risk factors for recurrent seizures include calcified brain lesions, multiple seizures, and multiple brain cysts (37). Steroids are commonly used to manage peri-cystic inflammation. It is always used with anthelmintics. Surgery in the management of neurocysticercosis is limited to managing hydrocephalus through CSF diversion, establishing a diagnosis via stereotactic biopsy or occasionally removal of a giant cyst that is causing neuronal compression or ventricular obstruction by endoscopic or open microsurgery.

Echinococcus

Echinococcus, also known as hydatid disease, is due to an infection by E. Granulosa, a dog tapeworm. This tapeworm is around 2–5 mm in length and uses sheep and man as its intermediate host (38). E. Granulosa infects humans through direct contact with dogs or by eating food contaminated with E. Granulosa eggs. When the eggs enter the human body, they hatch to form embryos which can burrow through the duodenal wall to gain spread through the body via a haematogenous route. The liver, lung and brain are common sites for the cyst to form (38). CNS involvement occurs in 3% of all Echinococcus infections. Cysts are normally located in the white matter, they can be solitary or multiple, but they do grow slowly. Symptoms arising from the cyst do not appear unless the cyst reaches a significant size to cause mass effect. Therefore, the symptoms arising from a hydatid cyst comprises of raised ICP, seizure, and focal neurological deficit. Enzyme-linked immunosorbent assay can help diagnose patients with Echinococcus.

Radiologically, the cyst is of similar characteristics to CSF. The cyst itself does not enhance but the surrounding parenchyma can enhance slightly due to perilesional inflammation (39). The cyst can contain multiple protoscolexes which, when ruptures, can cause the formation of multiple cysts in the surrounding tissue or allergic reactions. The management of echinococcus consists of anthelmintic therapy, such as Albendazole and surgery. The aim of surgery is to remove as the cyst with its content intact. Care must be taken while raising the craniotomy and performing the durotomy. Bipolar coagulation should be kept to a minimum, and the cyst wall should be kept moist to prevent rupture. Hydro-dissection using a rubber catheter within the lesion-brain plane can allow careful separation of the cyst from the surrounding brain. If the cyst ruptures, immediately suction up any cyst content and remove the capsule. The lesion cavity must then be washed thoroughly, and all instruments, gloves, and gowns should be changed (40).

PITFALLS AND PEARLS

- Cryptococcosis is managed with antifungal agents but may occasionally require CSF diversion when there is raised ICP.
- Most of the symptoms and complications arising from neurocysticercosis are due to the perilesional inflammation. Management of this inflammation with steroids is paramount.
- Care must be taken when surgically removing Echinococcus Cyst, as rupture of the cyst can cause secondary spread of the infection to the surrounding tissues.

References

1. Helweg-Larsen J, Astradsson A, Richhall H, et al. Pyogenic brain abscess, a 15 year survey. *BMC Infect Dis*. 30 November 2012 ;12:332.
2. Hollin SA, Hayashi H, Gross SW. Intracranial abscesses of odontogenic origin. *Oral Surg Oral Med Oral Pathol*. March 1967;23(3):277–93.
3. Dupuis-Girod S, Giraud S, Decullier E, et al. Hemorrhagic hereditary telangiectasia (Rendu-Osler disease) and infectious diseases: An underestimated association. *Clin Infect Dis*. 15 March 2007;44(6):841–5.
4. Kao PT, Tseng HK, Liu CP, Su SC, Lee CM. Brain abscess: Clinical analysis of 53 cases. *J Microbiol Immunol Infect*. June 2003;36(2):129–36.
5. Darlow CA, McGlashan N, Kerr R, et al. Microbial aetiology of brain abscess in a UK cohort: Prominent role of Streptococcus intermedius. *J Infect*. 2020;80(6):623–9.
6. Li X, Tronstad L, Olsen I. Brain abscesses caused by oral infection. *Endod Dent Traumatol*. June 1999;15(3):95–101.
7. Weerakkody RM, Palangasinghe DR, Wadanambi S, Wijewikrama ES. 'Primary' nocardial brain abscess in a renal transplant patient. *BMC Res Notes*. 23 November 2015;8:701.
8. Britt RH, Enzmann DR, Yeager AS. Neuropathological and computerized tomographic findings in experimental brain abscess. *J Neurosurg*. 1981;55(4):590–603.
9. Lee TH, Chang WN, Su TM, et al. Clinical features and predictive factors of intraventricular rupture in patients who have bacterial brain abscesses. *J Neurol Neurosurg Psychiatry*. March 2007;78(3):303–9.
10. Cartes-Zumelzu FW, Stavrou I, Castillo M, et al. Diffusion-weighted imaging in the assessment of brain abscesses therapy. *AJNR Am J Neuroradiol*. September 2004;25(8):1310–7.
11. Luthra G, Parihar A, Nath K, et al. Comparative evaluation of fungal, tubercular, and pyogenic brain abscesses with conventional and diffusion MR imaging and proton MR spectroscopy. *AJNR Am J Neuroradiol*. August 2007;28(7):1332–8.
12. Arlotti M, Grossi P, Pea F, et al. Consensus document on controversial issues for the treatment of infections of the central nervous system: Bacterial brain abscesses. *Int J Infect Dis*. October 2010;14 Suppl 4:S79–92.
13. Rosenblum ML, Hoff JT, Norman D, Edwards MS, Berg BO. Nonoperative treatment of brain abscesses in selected high-risk patients. *J Neurosurg*. February 1980;52(2):217–25.

References

14. Mamelak AN, Mampalam TJ, Obana WG, Rosenblum ML. Improved management of multiple brain abscesses: A combined surgical and medical approach. *Neurosurgery*. January 1995;36(1):76–85; discussion 85–6.
15. Osborn MK, Steinberg JP. Subdural empyema and other suppurative complications of paranasal sinusitis. *Lancet Infect Dis*. January 2007;7(1):62–7.
16. Munusamy T, Dinesh SK. Delayed occurrence of escherichia coli subdural empyema following head injury in an elderly patient: A case report and literature review. *J Neurol Surg Rep*. July 2015;76(1):e79–82.
17. Critchley G, Strachan R. Postoperative subdural empyema caused by Propionibacterium acnes – A report of two cases. *Br J Neurosurg*. June 1996;10(3):321–3.
18. Cowie R, Williams B. Late seizures and morbidity after subdural empyema. *J Neurosurg*. April 1983;58(4):569–73.
19. French H, Schaefer N, Keijzers G, Barison D, Olson S. Intracranial subdural empyema: A 10-year case series. *Ochsner J*. 2014;14(2):188–94.
20. Kubik CS, Adams RD. Subdural empyema. *Brain*. 1943;66(1):18–42.
21. Weisberg L. Subdural empyema: Clinical and computed tomographic correlations. *Arch Neurol*. May 1986;43(5):497–500.
22. Wong AM, Zimmerman RA, Simon EM, Pollock AN, Bilaniuk LT. Diffusion-weighted MR imaging of subdural empyemas in children. *AJNR Am J Neuroradiol*. 25(6):1016–21.
23. Mauser HW, Ravijst RA, Elderson A, van Gijn J, Tulleken CA. Nonsurgical treatment of subdural empyema: Case report. *J Neurosurg*. July 1985;63(1):128–30.
24. Leys D, Destee A, Petit H, Warot P. Management of subdural intracranial empyemas should not always require surgery. *J Neurol Neurosurg Psychiatry*. June 1986;49(6):635–9.
25. Bok AP, Peter JC. Subdural empyema: Burr holes or craniotomy? A retrospective computerized tomography-era analysis of treatment in 90 cases. *J Neurosurg*. April 1993;78(4):574–8.
26. Nathoo N, Nadvi SS, van Dellen JR. Cranial extradural empyema in the era of computed tomography: A review of 82 cases. *Neurosurgery*. April 1999;44(4):748–53; discussion 753–4.
27. Pradilla G, Ardila GP, Hsu W, Rigamonti D. Epidural abscesses of the CNS. *Lancet Neurol*. March 2009;8(3):292–300.
28. Weingarten K, Zimmerman RD, Becker RD, et al. Subdural and epidural empyemas: MR imaging. *AJR Am J Roentgenol*. March 1989;152(3):615–21.
29. Tsuchiya K, Osawa A, Katase S, et al. Diffusion-weighted MRI of subdural and epidural empyemas. *Neuroradiology*. April 2003;45(4):220–3.

30. Mitchell TG, Perfect JR. Cryptococcosis in the era of AIDS–100 years after the discovery of Cryptococcus neoformans. *Clin Microbiol Rev.* October 1995;8(4):515–48.
31. Kaplan JE, Benson C, Holmes KK, et al. Guidelines for prevention and treatment of opportunistic infections in HIV-infected adults and adolescents: Recommendations from CDC, the National Institutes of Health, and the HIV Medicine Association of the Infectious Diseases Society of America. *MMWR Recomm Rep.* 10 April 2009;58(RR-4):1–207; quiz CE1-4.
32. CDC. DPDx – Laboratory identification of parasites of public health concern. 2019 [cited 4 September 2022]. Cysticercosis. www.cdc.gov/dpdx/cysticercosis/index.html.
33. Garcia HH, Del Brutto OH, Cysticercosis Working Group in Peru. Neurocysticercosis: Updated concepts about an old disease. *Lancet Neurol.* October 2005;4(10):653–61.
34. Tsang VC, Brand JA, Boyer AE. An enzyme-linked immunoelectrotransfer blot assay and glycoprotein antigens for diagnosing human cysticercosis (Taenia solium). *J Infect Dis.* January 1989;159(1):50–9.
35. Mitchell WG, Crawford TO. Intraparenchymal cerebral cysticercosis in children: Diagnosis and treatment. *Pediatrics.* July 1988;82(1):76–82.
36. Del Brutto OH, Santibañez R, Noboa CA, et al. Epilepsy due to neurocysticercosis: Analysis of 203 patients. *Neurology.* February 1992;42(2):389–92.
37. Del Brutto OH. Prognostic factors for seizure recurrence after withdrawal of antiepileptic drugs in patients with neurocysticercosis. *Neurology.* September 1994;44(9):1706–9.
38. Brunetti E, White AC. Cestode infestations: Hydatid disease and cysticercosis. *Infect Dis Clin North Am.* June 2012;26(2):421–35.
39. Abdel Razek AAK, El-Shamam O, Abdel Wahab N. Magnetic resonance appearance of cerebral cystic echinococcosis: World Health Organization (WHO) classification. *Acta Radiol.* June 2009;50(5):549–54.
40. Carrea R, Dowling E, Guevara JA. Surgical treatment of hydatid cysts of the central nervous system in the pediatric age (Dowling's technique). *Childs Brain.* 1975;1(1):4–21.

Cambridge Elements

Emergency Neurosurgery

Nihal Gurusinghe
Lancashire Teaching Hospital NHS Trust

Professor Nihal Gurusinghe is a Consultant Neurosurgeon at the Lancashire Teaching Hospitals NHS Trust. He is on the Executive Council of the Society of British Neurological Surgeons as the Lead for NICE (National Institute for Health and Care Excellence) guidelines relating to neurosurgical practice. He is also an examiner for the UK and International FRCS examinations in Neurosurgery.

Peter Hutchinson
University of Cambridge, Society of British Neurological Surgeons and Royal College of Surgeons of England

Peter Hutchinson BSc MBBS FFSEM FRCS(SN) PhD FMedSci is Professor of Neurosurgery and Head of the Division of Academic Neurosurgery at the University of Cambridge, and Honorary Consultant Neurosurgeon at Addenbrooke's Hospital. He is Director of Clinical Research at the Royal College of Surgeons of England and Meetings Secretary of the Society of British Neurological Surgeons.

Ioannis Fouyas
Royal College of Surgeons of Edinburgh

Ioannis Fouyas is a Consultant Neurosurgeon in Edinburgh. His clinical interests focus on the treatment of complex cerebrovascular and skull base pathologies. His academic endeavours concentrate in the field of cerebrovascular pathophysiology. His passion is technical surgical training, fulfilled in collaboration with the Royal College of Surgeons of Edinburgh. Finally, he pursues Undergraduate Neuroscience teaching, with a particular focus on functional Neuroanatomy.

Naomi Slator
North Bristol NHS Trust

Naomi Slator FRCS (SN) is a Consultant Spinal Neurosurgeon based at North Bristol NHS Trust. She has a specialist interest in Complex Spine alongside Cranial and Spinal Trauma. She completed her neurosurgical training in Birmingham and a six-month Fellowship in CSF and Trauma (2019). She then went on to complete her Spinal Fellowship in Leeds (2020) before moving to the southwest to take up her consultant post.

Ian Kamaly-Asl
Royal Manchester Children's Hospital

Ian Kamaly-Asl is a full time paediatric neurosurgeon and Honorary Chair at Royal Manchester Children's Hospital. He trained in North Western Deanery with fellowships at Boston Children's Hospital and Sick Kids in Toronto. Ian is a member of council of The Royal College of Surgeons of England and The SBNS where he is lead for mentoring and tackling oppressive behaviours.

Peter Whitfield
University Hospitals Plymouth NHS Trust

Professor Peter Whitfield is a Consultant Neurosurgeon at the South West Neurosurgical Centre, University Hospitals Plymouth NHS Trust. His clinical interests include vascular neurosurgery, neuro oncology and trauma. He has held many roles in postgraduate neurosurgical education and is President of the Society of British Neurological Surgeons. Peter has published widely, and is passionate about education, training and the promotion of clinical research.

About the Series

Elements in Emergency Neurosurgery is intended for trainees and practitioners in Neurosurgery and Emergency Medicine as well as allied specialties all over the world. Authored by international experts, this series provides core knowledge, common clinical pathways and recommendations on the management of acute conditions of the brain and spine.

Cambridge Elements

Emergency Neurosurgery

Elements in the Series

Spinal Discitis and Epidural Abscess
Damjan Veljanoski and Pragnesh Bhatt

Adult Patient with Intraventricular, Paraventricular and Pineal Region Lesions
Mohamed Dablouk and Mahmoud Kamel

Ruptured Supratentorial Cerebral Artery Aneurysm with Large Intracerebral Haematoma
Samuel Hall and Diederik Bulters

Neurosurgical Handovers and Standards for Emergency Care
Simon Lammy and Jennifer Brown

Spontaneous Intracranial Haemorrhage Caused by a Non-aneurysmal Brain Vascular Malformation
Sherif R. W. Kirollos and Ramez W. Kirollos

Emergency Scenarios in Functional Neurosurgery
James Manfield and Nicholas Park

Management of a Patient with a Venous Sinus Thrombosis with or without an Intracerebral Haematoma
Helen Sims and James Choulerton

Patient with Suspected Cauda Equina Syndrome
Gabriel Metcalf-Cuenca and Patrick F. X. Statham

Patient with Acute Thoracic Myelopathy due to Degenerative Disease
James M. W. Robins and Deb Pal

Management of Moderate or Severe Traumatic Brain Injury
Saeed Kayhanian, Erta Beqiri, Ari Ercole and Adel Helmy

Assessment of a Patient in Coma
Alexander Shah and Holly Roy

Intracranial Abscess in Adults
See Yung Phang and William Taylor

A full series listing is available at: www.cambridge.org/EEMN

For EU product safety concerns, contact us at Calle de José Abascal, 56–1°, 28003 Madrid, Spain or eugpsr@cambridge.org.

www.ingramcontent.com/pod-product-compliance
Ingram Content Group UK Ltd.
Pitfield, Milton Keynes, MK11 3LW, UK
UKHW021615130126
466887UK00018B/247